# Wicca
# for
# Beginners

*A complete guide to start practicing with magical spells and rituals using Wiccan herbs, candles and crystals, moon cycles and more, which will lead you to change your lifestyle, increasing your personal power.*

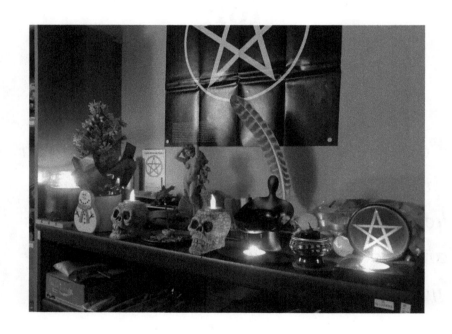

# Table of Contents

# Introduction

Congratulations on downloading *Wicca for Beginners* and thank you for doing so.

The following chapters will discuss everything that you'll need to know as a witch who's just starting out. We will dive into the ancient history of Paganism on which Wicca was founded, the modern history of Wicca in the 20th century, and the current state of the religion today.

This work will also dive into the divine archetypes worshipped in Wicca, with a special focus on the Lord and Lady, also known as the Triple Goddess and the Horned God. We will also have a brief overview of other deities sometimes worshipped in the Wiccan system. There will also be a chapter that describes the four elements and their meanings, and how you can use them to cast a magical circle.

There are many tools that are very important to this religion, such as the athame, the wand, the chalice, and the pentacle. We will dive into the symbolism of each of these tools, as well as how they can be placed on altars, and how they can be used in rituals. We will explore how those rituals take place on sacred festivals, as well as during the full moon.

Finally, this book will explore the use of magic, and the recording of spells in a personal Book of Shadows, as well as how to grow your practice as either a solitary practitioner or a member of a coven.

There are plenty of books on this subject on the market, thanks again for choosing this one! Every effort was made to ensure it is full of as much useful information as possible, please enjoy!

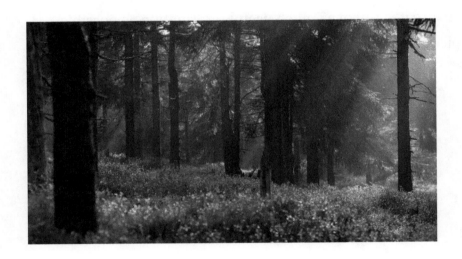

# Summer

For most people, summer begins Memorial Day weekend. On official government calendars, it begins on June 21st. For the ancients, however, summer began on May 1st, with the fire festival of Beltane. Summer was a favorite time of year in the ancient world because life was easy. There was hard work to be done in the fields, but the natural world was providing everything that they needed to survive. Berries were ripening, wild game was fattening up from the long winter, and new livestock was being born.

During this time, the deer are growing new antlers. You can see the velvety nubs on their heads growing slowly as the season progresses. The small animals have completely grown up; the rabbits have left the warren, and the songbirds have fledged and left the nests. The babies of the larger animals, such as deer, foxes, and wolves, have begun to enter adolescence and are learning how to survive from their mothers. The plants have shed their springtime flowers and are now sporting rich green leaves; many are also actively producing fruit or putting effort into doing so by the time that the autumn rolls around. It is a time of warmth, growth, learning, and maturing.

Summer is the part of the year that corresponds with young adulthood in the cycle of human life. The summer is the "prime" of the year; similarly, young adulthood is when we are in the "prime." The sun is at the height of its power and the Earth is at the height of its growth and prosperity. Similarly, humans during this phase have strong bodies that are able to accomplish many amazing feats, and they have amazing amounts of energy to go out and accomplish their dreams. This is one of the most energetic times of the year, with animals feasting in order to put on weight for the winter. Young adulthood is also one of the most energetic times of someone's life, as they go out in the world and attempt to figure out who they are.

During this time of year, there was an astounding amount of feasting that happened in ancient times. Because this was the season of plenty, there was no starvation, and the days were long. There was finally time to enjoy life. Even though there was a massive amount of work to be done intending the fields, once the day's work was done, our ancestors lit fires and took lovers down to the woods. This time of year was the height of work, but also the height of pleasure. The work largely consisted of weeding the fields, watering them to ensure the young plants grew to their full height and tending to livestock to ensure that the herds stayed strong, healthy, and well-fed.

If you are performing spell work in which you are trying to effect changes out in the physical world, summer is the best season in which to do it. In correspondence with the principles of yin and yang, winter is yin, or the still, quiet, and receptive season. Summer is the yang season: it is full of action, power, and movement. You can tap into that power to cause change. The sun is also at its fullest power on the summer solstice; you can tap into the powerful, manifesting power of the sun's fire, and use that energy in your spell work. Manifestation is associated with the element of fire; the summer is also associated with the element of fire. Use this fiery power to manifest those things in your life which you most need. However, it is also necessary to exercise extreme contemplation, restraint, and discernment when attempting to harness so much fiery energy. As previously stated, fire can burn. And in the case of manifesting your desires, be sure that you really want what you are attempting to summon to your life; after all, you just might get it.

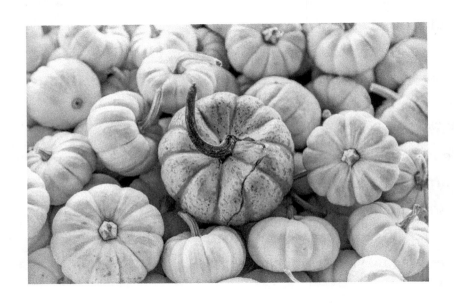

# Fall

Today, most people associate autumn with apple cider and pumpkin spice lattes. When the leaves begin to fall, many people rush out to take photos of the many different colored tree leaves. For the ancients, though, fall was the beginning of a time of fear. The days were starting to shorten, and the looming shadow of winter appeared. Like squirrels, our ancestors furiously put away stores for the winter, knowing that the amount of food they put away would be the only thing standing between them and starvation.

The most noticeable thing that happens during this season is the changing of the leaves. The turn vibrant red, orange, or yellow, and begin to drop. There are more subtle signs too, though. The last of the fruits are beginning to ripen on the branch and on the vine. The days have reached equal length, and soon the nights will be longer than the days, signaling the descent into the dark season of winter. The behaviors of the animals have also begun to change. Those who will stay through the winter are fattening up in order to ensure they will have stores to make it through the cold season. Those that will not stay begin to migrate away. Everyone is familiar with the great V's of geese that begin to head south for the winter.

This part of the year is associated with middle age in the human life cycle. Just as the natural world has begun to lose the vibrancy and vigor of summer, so too do people at this age begin to lose the physical prowess and vibrancy of youth. The natural world is also putting out prodigious amounts of fruit and bounty. Similarly, people who have reached this age have begun to metaphorically harvest the lessons of their life and to turn their experiences into valuable wisdom and resources for their communities. While this season may not have the ease of summer, it is when the true work of one's life begins to bear fruit.

This time of year is excellent for spells to help you maintain stamina to the end of the finish line. If you are running low on energy and trying to complete a project or idea that you have long labored on, you can tap into the magic of this time of year in order to help your project bear fruit. You can also use the energy of the natural world to gain insight as to what you should be harvesting from your life. This time of year is an excellent opportunity to review the lessons of your life and metaphorically "harvest" the wisdom that you might find there.

# Winter

The modern day has robbed winter of the worst of its bite. People get cold, but they can retreat into heated houses, put hand-warmers inside their gloves, and get where they need to go inside of heated automobiles. It is only when the power goes out in the middle of a blizzard that people begin to feel a twinge of what our ancestors felt in the face of the coldest season. They huddled together around great hearths for warmth, carefully rationing out their stores, hoping that they would last until spring. With so many people so close together, illness and sickness spread easily during this time.

The natural world is blanketed in stillness. If you have ever wandered out in the middle of a snowstorm, you'll notice that the world is eerily quiet. It's as if the entire landscape has become hushed; there is no movement, and it is easy to believe that you are the only creature or person in the world. This season is the height of yin energy or stillness. It is the time for receptivity, for meditation and turning inward. All of the animals are hidden in their burrows hibernating or have flown south for the winter. There are very few animals that are active during this time. You may see the flash of fox hunting, or catch a glimpse of a squirrel digging up a cache of nuts it stored earlier that year. For the most part, though, all of the animals have gone to ground. The only thing that is still green is the pine trees. Their tough needles ensure that they can stay green even in the deepest cold. To our ancestors, those evergreen trees were symbols of the greenery that would return with the spring, which is why they brought sprigs of them inside.

This time of year equates with old age and death in the human life cycle. Just as the world has gone quiet and still, so too in old age do we slow down. The world enters into a meditative state, and old age provides us with the opportunity to reflect on the experiences of our lives. Just as our ancient ancestors gathered around hearth fires in the winter and told stories, so too does old age provide us the opportunity to connect with our communities and share the wisdom that we have gathered over the course of our lives. In olden times, elders were venerated and held in high regard, because the wisdom that they held in their living memory was a valuable resource for those trying to figure out the best ways to live their lives.

This was the time of waiting for our ancestors. They would ration their stores and hope that the food they had put away would last until the spring thaw. It was a time when the fear of starvation was very real. Because people were so close together in such cramped quarters, people grew ill very easily. It was a hard time. However, it was also a time of storytelling and communal gathering. It was the time when the community came together from their scattered summer wanderings and duties and forged strong clan and tribal ties. It is these ties that united them as a people.

If you are lost and seeking wisdom in your life, winter is an excellent time to perform magic to seek the wisdom of your ancestors. It is also a great time to perform restorative magic. Winter is the meditative season. This season is a wonderful opportunity to gather energy in preparation for the work of the coming year.

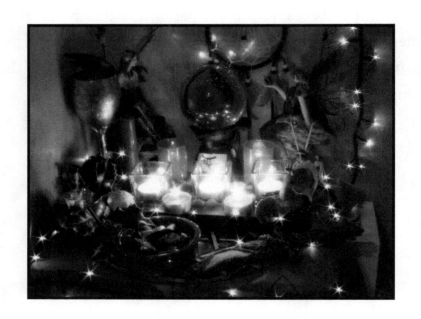

# Chapter 1 : Sabbats

In Wicca, sabbats are the celebrations that occur throughout the year, and which coincide with the changing of the seasons as well as the equinoxes. As a nature-based faith, Wiccan practitioners mark their days in conjunction with the natural world, recognizing and celebrating the ebb and flow of life in all things.

The sabbats also follow the mythical stories of the god and the goddess: at Yule, the Oak King (or Sun god) is born, and he grows quietly towards adolescence throughout the winter. At springtime, he and the goddess are young adults, joining together to bring life back to the Earth at Beltane, the sabbat observed on the first of May. At the height of summer, when Litha is celebrated, the Oak King has reached maturity, and soon after he declines, giving his body to the Earth at Lammas so that the harvest may be bountiful. At Litha/midsummer, the Holly King is born—a mirror opposite of the Oak King, and he grows to maturity until, at Yule and the darkest night, he succumbs to old age as well to nourish the sleeping animals and plants beneath the mantle of winter's snow and ice.

# Yule

Yule occurs on the winter solstice, between December 20th and 23rd. It is known as the shortest day of the year, as well as the darkest night, for those living in the Northern hemisphere.

At Samhain, we began to sense that the Veil—the wall between the living world and the spiritual world—was opening. Picture a curtain in a theater slowly becoming transparent, until it's gone. That's what's happening after the Oak King passes into the Earth at the end of summer, culminating at Yule. This is a time for reflection, remembrance, and most importantly— survival. When the Veil is gone, the gods and goddesses are busy, attending to their affairs. They haven't completely left humanity's side and you can still pray to them, but they are voices in the dark of winter, far away.

That is why at Yule; we gather close and celebrate community because the community is what enabled our ancestors to survive the cold, dark winter.

**The rebirth of the Sun.** On this night, the slow return of the sun is celebrated. Wiccans carry on the traditions of the ancestors when crops and trees were blessed with cider, called *wassail*, and wine and gifts of the harvest's fruits were given from house to house. In some countries, a tradition of giving books continues to this day. Rituals to cheer the spirit and keep the dark at bay, such as the lighting of candles and bonfires, are also practiced in modern times.

**Symbols of Yule.** Mistletoe, holly, the adorning of evergreen trees—thought to be aspects of the divine by Celtic peoples— are all originally pagan symbols and used to decorate homes and altars during this sabbat. Additionally, the **yule log** was used to celebrate the rebirth of the Sun god, using a small piece of last year's log to set this year's ablaze after it's been decorated with pine, blessed with wine or cider, and sprinkled with flour—the representation of the mingling of the god and goddess.

**Gods and Goddesses of Yule:** Any sun gods and mother goddesses, as well as triple goddesses. Fire goddesses such as Brigid.

**Herbs:** thistle, frankincense, rosemary, sage, laurel, bay.

**Foods:** wassail, liquor-soaked cakes, roasted game meats or pork, turkey, bread.

**Colors of Yule:** gold, green, silver, white, and red.

**Crystals:** Herkimer diamond, bloodstone, agate, pyrite, amber, emerald.

**Appropriate spell work:** Anything to do with love, friendship, rekindling, inspiration, warmth, and comfort. Yule is a good time to focus on the positive and reaffirm one's self.

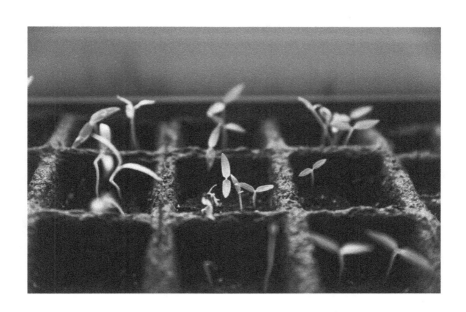

# Imbolc

Also known as Candlemas and St. Brigid's Day, Imbolc is celebrated on February 2nd. It celebrates the first, inspirational spark that happens when we feel the hidden life beneath the frozen soil stir. The word "Imbolc" means "in the mother's belly", and so can we consider the sleeping seeds and hibernating animals at this time, in Earth's womb. Another name for this sabbat was Olneic, meaning "ewe's milk", dating back to traditional lambing season. On Imbolc, we celebrate the hope of life during the middle mark of winter.

The maiden goddess is celebrated at this time, and the sabbat is particularly auspicious of Brigid, the Celtic goddess of fire, poetry, blacksmithing, midwifery, and inspiration. The proper pronunciation of Brigid is the *bride*, and new brides and maidens are held in great regard on this day. Corn dollies and Brigid's crosses made of corn leaves are made to decorate the altar and give as gifts.

At this time of year, it's a good practice to symbolically sweep out last year's energy with a besom, in order to sweep in the new. Crocuses are a symbol of the maiden goddess, testing the air to see if spring is close by. Light a candle in each room to celebrate the goddess; go on walks in the snow to recognize and celebrate the first stirrings of spring.

**A time of inspiration and dedication.** This is a time when promises are made, devotions are set forth, and dedications to a new path are inscribed. New beginnings, reaffirmation of unions, and wiccanings (name-giving of children) are often celebrated and focused on.

**Symbols of Imbolc.** White flowers, candles, Brigid's crosses, copper, acorn-tipped wands to symbolize the sun god coming to adolescence, candle-crowns.

**Goddesses of Imbolc:** In addition to Brigid, this day is also the feast-day (birthday) of the Yoruban goddess Oya, who represents fire, lightning, the rainbow, the beloved dead, and the marketplace.

**Herbs:** violets, vervain, basil, angelica.

**Foods:** dairy, herbal tea, seeded cakes, roasted sunflower and pumpkin seeds, greens.

**Colors of Imbolc:** white, pale green, yellow, pink, red.

**Crystals:** white quartz, citrine, amethyst, garnet, onyx.

**Appropriate spell work:** Reunion, renewal, commitment, planting the seeds of tomorrow.

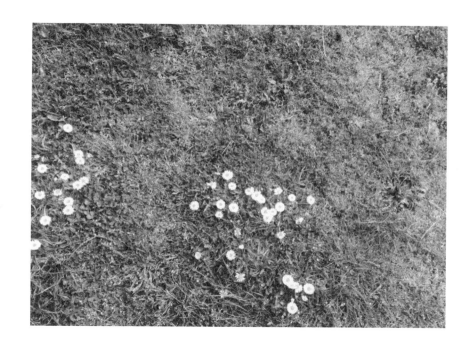

# Ostara – The Spring Equinox

The vernal equinox arrives between March 20th and 23rd, and on Ostara, we celebrate the fertility of the goddess in mother form. The ancient symbols of the egg and the hare are connected to the goddess Eostre, from which the word estrogen is derived.

At this time, the Sun god has also reached sexual maturity and enters into holy marriage with the goddess. Altars are decorated with symbols of fertility, as well as a chalice and athame, to symbolize the physical union of god and goddess.

Mythically, in nine months, the mother goddess will give birth to the harvest itself as well as the Oak King at Yule, in December. At this time, we give thanks for what we can expect to come to fruition in our futures, and for the ongoing fertility of the Earth.

At this time of year, we can see greater evidence of spring, and decorate our altars and homes with dyed eggs (preferably with natural dyes such as beetroot, tea, thistle, and other plants), and symbols of the hare.

**A time of planting.** Seedlings can be started indoors now, and the seeds of future endeavors marked by spell work and dedication, also. Plan a magical herb garden, and spend time out of doors breathing in the scents of new life.

**Symbols of Ostara.** Eggs, hares, baby animals, plants and flowers, pregnant mothers.

**Gods and Goddesses of Ostara:** All mother goddesses and fertility gods. Also Artemis, goddess of the hunt, Pan, the sun god Lugh, and the Horned God.

**Herbs and flowers:** ginger, frankincense, copal, chamomile, chickweed, iris, daffodils.

**Foods:** similar to Imbolc: herbal tea, seeded cakes, leafy dishes and dishes with flowers. Dairy dishes.

**Colors of Ostara:** green, yellow, lavender, white.

**Crystals:** amethyst, jasper, bloodstone.

**Appropriate spell work:** Prosperity, fertility, creativity, new endeavors.

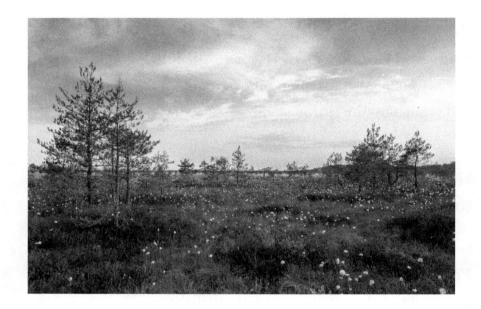

# Beltane

Celebrated either on the eve of April 30th or the day of May 1st, Beltane celebrates the union of the god and goddess as lovers and the death of winter. In high spring, hearts and minds focus on the coming summer, and easier days full of life and abundance. Beltane gets its name in part from Belinos, an ancient god of fire. Traditions of Beltane include community bonfires, feasts, and Maypoles. This is the second time of the year when the veil between the worlds is thin, and we may feel unrest and change unfurling within us, often giving way to vivid dreams.

Ancient practices allowed established married couples to leave their wedding bands at home for this night; younger people would camp in the woods and arrive home by the morning to participate in the Maypole dances. The morning of May 1st is especially magical for water spells: dew, rainwater, and river water collected at that time may be used for luck and fertility magic.

At this time of year, it's a good practice give yourself permission to enjoy life to the fullest—whichever way that means for you, as long as it does no harm. Realize that even the most docile, quiet creature is permitted to kick up its heels sometimes. You are doing nothing more but celebrating the joy of being alive, in the name of the god and goddess.

**A time of community.** Many Wiccan solitary practitioners choose to come out for Beltane, whether it's to join others in a potluck feast, sit by a roaring bonfire, or join together to perform a traditional Maypole dance. It is a happy, festive time for all ages.

**Symbols of Beltane.** White flowers, candles, Brigid's crosses, copper, acorn-tipped wands to symbolize the sun god coming to adolescence, candle-crowns.

**Gods and Goddesses of Beltane:** Bacchus, Cernunnos, Hera, Pan, Sheela-Na-Gig, Oshun, Yemaya, Corn Woman. In addition, the faerie and nature spirits can be connected to at this time.

**Herbs and flowers:** hyacinth, lilac, rose, basil, oregano, and cinquefoil.

**Foods:** almonds and nuts, apples, vanilla-flavored cakes, Meade, oysters, fresh greens.

**Colors of Beltane:** orange, red, white, spring green, purple.

**Crystals:** bloodstone, hematite, rubies, tiger's eye, amber.

**Appropriate spell work:** Fertility, abundance, money-related magic, love blessings.

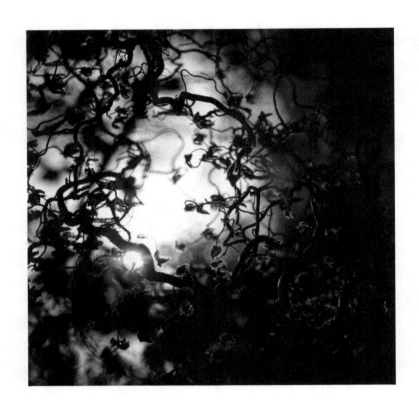

# Litha

The summer solstice occurs between June 20th and June 22nd, and this is the longest day of the year. This marks the height of power of the god, and the Green Man—a Briton god of the forest and whose ivy-wreathed face is found in many ancient churches to this day—is in his glory. Midsummer Eve is auspiciously connected to the faerie realm, and dishes of milk and honey are set beneath oak trees for the fae folk, in appreciation for their hard work of wild animal husbandry and tending the plants and flowers of summer.

In the midst of summer's abundance and life, there is a deeper meaning to Litha: the Oak King is doing battle with the Holly King, who will return to Earth soon to rule the darkening days until Yule. There is a power struggle between life and death, darkness and light. This is a good time to resolve conflicts within yourself and do magical work seeking to incorporate our shadows (natural qualities of ourselves we might be uncomfortable with) and make peace within our spirits.

While harvest is not yet here, Litha is still a good time to take stock of the blessings in your life and be thankful for what you have. Use this time to focus on life's joys, and strive to be in the moment as you celebrate them.

**A time of sunlight and fertility.** Fertility not only pertains to having children. For the artist, entrepreneur, or anyone who works with their hands, fertility means promise, innate talents, and the power to take raw talent and be successful at one's vocation. Be thankful for the gifts you've been blessed with. Make pacts to work hard to bring them to their highest peak. Thank the Sun god for his life-giving warmth at this time. Re-dedicate yourself to the god and goddess.

**Symbols of Litha.** Horned animals, the oak tree, flowers, fresh water, the wand, and the crown.

**Gods and Goddesses of Litha:** Herne (a woodland god), Lugh, Pan, the Green Man, Amaterasu (a Japanese Shinto goddess of the sun), Hestia (goddess of the hearth).

**Herbs and Flowers:** goldenrod, honeysuckle, jasmine, sunflower, vervain, mug wort, oak, elder, lemon verbena.

**Foods:** sweet cakes, dandelion wine, meade, foraged foods, eggs, freshwater fish, oatcakes, cheeses, honey.

**Colors of Litha:** forest green, pink, yellow, brown.

**Crystals:** emerald, peridot, chrysoprase, agate, amber, opal.

**Appropriate spell work:** Conflict resolution, unity, abundance, gratitude.

# Lammas

Also known as Lughnasadh, Lammas is celebrated on August 1st and commemorates the death of the Oak King and the birth of the Holly King. Summer is dying and harvest has begun. The days will soon grow darker, but until then, we give thanks for the god's sacrifice; the Oak King gives his body to the Earth to ensure the harvest is bountiful enough for us to survive the winter.

Under the hot sun, plants brown and wither, releasing their seeds to the soil for next year. This is the link between the Oak King and the flora and fauna of the world.

Lammas in ancient times meant "loaf mass". It is traditional to give gifts of bread. Additionally, the craftsman god Lugh, also connected with the sun, bade us work hard and relish the fruits of our labors.

At this time of year, it's a good practice to take stock of what we have and to see how far we've come in our endeavors and goals. While winter is around the corner, right now the sun is hot, the tables are full, and so should our hearts be. Relish the beauty of the natural world and let it buoy your spirits.

**A time of abundance and honoring ancestors.** In modern times we often take for granted how easy it is to acquire food and nourishment. For our ancestors, this was the least idle time of year. A good harvest was crucial to survival. Pay homage to your ancestors, and perform healing magic on behalf of those in the world who still have to struggle for food. Donate to your local food pantries or volunteer at community kitchens.

**Symbols of Lammas.** White flowers, candles, Brigid's crosses, copper, acorn-tipped wands to symbolize the sun god coming to adolescence, candle-crowns.

**Gods of Lammas:** Lugh, sun gods, and the Holly King.

**Herbs and plants:** goldenrod, bloodroot, garlic, Queen Anne's lace, apple, wheat, bee balm, barley, mint, meadowsweet, thistle, nettle, rue.

**Foods:** dairy, herbal tea, seeded cakes, roasted sunflower and pumpkin seeds, greens.

**Colors of Lammas:** white, pale green, yellow, pink, red.

**Crystals:** white quartz, citrine, amethyst, garnet, onyx.

**Appropriate spell work:** Reunion, renewal, commitment, planting the seeds of tomorrow.

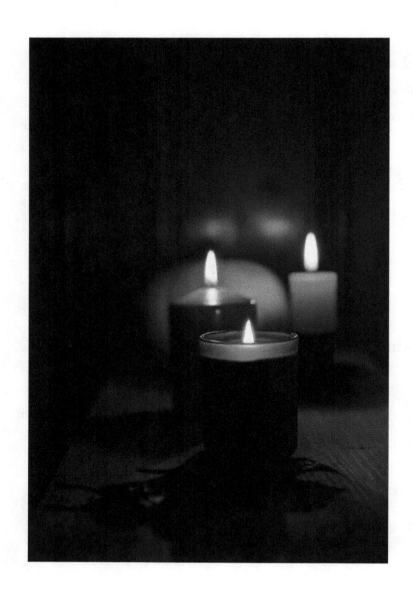

# Mabon

Mabon continues the harvest that began at Lammas. It is known as the second harvest and is a time to celebrate family, home, and hearth, as well as the fruits of our endeavors.

Mabon also begins the more somber of the sabbats, as this is the time that the goddess descends into the underworld, passing through the veil. The Earth begins to cool and the plants of the forest, farm, and field are withering. The forests begin to pay homage to the goddess by seeming to light themselves ablaze with color; a tribute from the god himself.

At this time of year, it's to focus on giving thanks for what you have. You may not be a gardener or a farmer, but you toil and put care into something—be it your career, your art, raising your children, caring for your pets, or simply living a peaceful, authentic life. Celebrate all of the days that led up to this one, in making you the person you are today.

**A time of thankfulness, and the celebration of elders.** Elders hold a special place in the Wiccan community. For everything they've shared with us—their wisdom, their hard work, their love—we elevate them and place importance on them during the Mabon feast. The goddess at this time in the year becomes the Crone, and her consort, the god, prepares himself for death and eventual rebirth. It is a quieting of the world as living things prepare for rest and to be reborn in spring.

**Symbols of Mabon.** Cornucopia, gourd rattles, corn and wheat, apples, pumpkins.

**Gods and Goddesses of Mabon:** Persephone and Hades, Snake Woman, Thor, Dionysus, Bacchus, Herne, the Muses, Loki.

**Herbs and plants:** copal, benzoin, frankincense, Solomon's seal, sage, milkweed, tobacco.

**Foods:** bread, vegetables harvested from the garden, roast meats, root vegetables, corn, apples, pomegranates.

**Colors of Mabon:** red, brown, orange, gold, white, and black.

**Crystals:** lapis, turquoise, yellow agate.

**Appropriate spell work:** rites of passage, family and connection, personal strength, abundance, removal of doubt.

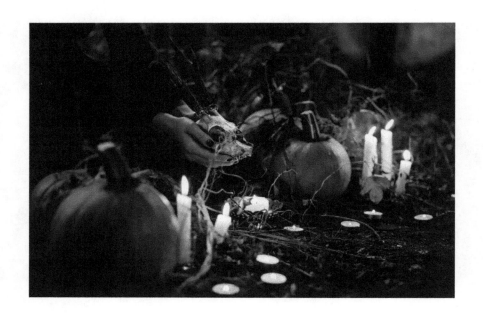

# Samhain

Arguably the most auspicious of the pagan holidays, Samhain (pronounced *sow*-when), marks the end of the year and the opening of the veil between the mortal world and the spiritual world. We honor our beloved dead and look upon the wheel of the year, as well as time itself, recognizing that death is not the end, but another place on the wheel. Life continues, and dark and light are simply part of the natural order of things.

Other names for Samhain are All Hallow's (or simply Hallows), Shadow fest (in Italian *Strega* witchcraft), and the Day of the Dead.

This time of year, we honor the goddess as Crone and the aged god as dark lord and lady. Darkness is not evil—it is a part of the natural world. Winter's days are shorter and the nights' darkness longer; death precedes birth and birth to death, and so forth turns the Wheel of the Year and of time itself.

At this time of year, we look to the spirit world with great care and empathy. We set places at the table, known as a mute supper, for the beloved dead. Our ancestors buried apples along the side of the road, set plates of food out on the doorstep, and hollowed out turnips to place candles into light the way of the dead to warm fires and loving hearts.

**A time of reverence.** This time of year, we honor all who have passed before us, as well as the god and goddess for all of the life they've given us in the year. We look at our own growth, and make vows for change or for courage, vows for love and for peace. We gather with our loved ones and reach out to our beloved dead to let them know that they will never be forgotten.

**Symbols of Samhain.** Pomegranate, apple, iron, cauldrons, besoms, jack-o-lanterns.

**Gods and Goddesses of Samhain:** Hecate, Oya (she also rules the cemetery), Isis, Baba Yaga, Rhiannon, the Morrigan, Lilith, Cerridwen, Kali, Hel, Ishtar. Hades, Ogun (Yoruban god of the forest and the forge), Anubis, Osiris, Cernunnos, Dionysus.

**Herbs:** mug wort, allspice, Mandrake, broom, sage, myrrh.

**Foods:** turnips, pumpkin, dark greens, baked bread, red wine, beef and pork, poultry, sweet cakes, and candies.

**Colors of Samhain:** orange and red, black, white, gold, and silver.

**Crystals:** jet, obsidian, onyx, iron, tiger's eye, white quartz.

# Chapter 2: Esbats

## What Is Moon Magic?

Humans have worshipped the moon and the sun for as long as there have been humans on Earth. Sometimes the moon is considered a male force of nature, and as such, the waxing moon is connected to the horned god, the full moon linked with the Fatherly aspect of the god, and the waning moon considered the elder god and the teacher.

More often, the moon is considered a planetary body that exists within the goddess's domain. The human menstrual cycle is typically 28 to 30 days, and so is the lunar cycle—the time it takes for the moon to travel around our Earth. The full moon is considered to be the fertile, motherly goddess, the waxing moon the maiden, and the waning moon the wise Crone.

Additionally, each full moon that occurs within a year—twelve to thirteen occurrences—has a name or special significance in many of the world's cultures, such as the native tribes of the

Americas and Canada, the Irish people, and West African tribes.

When two full moons fall in the same month, the second full moon is known as a *blue moon*, and special celebrations and magic may be performed during this time.

**The shifting moon.** The phases of the moon and the corresponding full moons will always shift slightly against the solar calendar. This coincides beautifully with the nature of the moon itself—in magic and in Wicca, the moon represents deep mysteries and ancient wisdom, and the fact that not everything in life is obvious or easy to come by. The moon takes patience and a serene mind to understand, and it takes time. The moon teaches us that life is a lesson—so it's useless to rush certain things when only time will bring them to us.

**The cleansing and rejuvenating power of the moon.** Something pagans often do is lay out there magical tools and crystals to recharge beneath the light of the full moon (even if that full moon reaches peak fullness during the middle of the day). The moon's energy washes us in potent power, full of promise and fertility. The triple goddess has been worshipped for thousands of years, in many different cultures, and has always been linked to the three phases of the moon.

**The moon and the phases of life.** For everything, there is a purpose and a meaning. As the moon shifts from crescent, to full, to opposite crescent, so do we focus our magical work on the moon's phase at the time.

# The New Moon Esbat

The word *esbat* comes from the same Greek origins as the word *estru* and means monthly". Some covens and communities choose to have their monthly esbat during the new moon. This moon can be a time to work with either the maiden goddess or the crone. It is a time of dark energy—and again, dark in pagan faiths does not mean evil, it simply means of the darkness. The night is dark and so is the womb. Onyx and crow's feathers are dark, and so is the soil. So don't fear the dark! It is a time of potency—consider it a blank canvas.

During a new moon esbat, the altar can be decorated with things reflecting the new moon's energy:

- Items that represent the maiden such as flower buds and seeds, a cup of soil, moonstones, crystal, a silver cord, a crow's feather; items that represent the crone such as a bundle of dried herbs (rosemary is perfect for this), a cup of sand or ashes, black coffee, onyx, turquoise, or beryl, an owl's feather.

- A statue or painting of either the maiden or the crone.

- Brown, dark purple, dark red or black candles.

- A besom, or sacred broom, to sweep away negative energy.

- The usual magical tools: chalice, athame, wand, and pentacle.

- An offering for the goddess, such as a cup of fresh water, bread, candied ginger, white wine, or grape juice. Typically, one beverage and one food are given. These can be passed around the circle for each to take a small part of before offering it to the goddess, and the person passing this to each member will say as they do so, "Never hunger, never thirst." This blesses each for the coming month.

During a new moon esbat, one may focus on cleansing a space or one's self of negative energies. Esbats can be celebrated alone or within a group. If solitary, a ritual cleansing bath, smudging (using sage, rosemary, or palo santo to burn cleansing smoke) a house or living area, or lighting a black candle followed by a white candle are all effective, simple cleansing techniques. Writing something you want to be rid of, such as a habit, guilt, grief, or shame, can be written on a piece of paper and burned in honor of the moon.

Once the cleansing is complete, a blessing should follow. Always follow the bitter with the sweet. Light sweet incense, draw the power of the potent moon's potential into your space, and shake bouquets of sweet flowers with holy water or rainwater around the circle and on the altar. Ask the goddess to bless the coming days of the month with sweetness and joy.

Once all ritual is complete, thank the goddess or god for joining your circle and celebrate with the traditional pagan "cakes and ale". This can be any combination of food and drink and doesn't have to include alcoholic beverages.

# The Waxing Moon Esbat

During a waxing moon esbat, the altar can be decorated in such a way as to honor the maiden.

- Items that represent the maiden, such as fresh milk, spring or rainwater, new flowers, white quartz, found bird feathers, nuts and seeds, ceramic statues of birds or young animals, citrine, peridot, moonstones, and tiger's eye.

- A statue or painting of maiden.

- White, silver, gray, or pale green or pale brown candles.

- The usual magical tools: chalice, athame, wand, and pentacle.

- An offering for the goddess, such as a cup of fresh water, honeyed cakes, crackers or cookies, white sparkling grape juice or white wine.

During a waxing moon esbat, spell work and rituals involving beginnings, courage, and hope, starting a project, new love, and life's milestones may be conducted.

During the waxing moon, we can focus our meditations and magical work on things we want to see come to fruition. Projects we are beginning, or have been working on, hopes of fertility, new relationships, and a new goal— all of these are well-suited to focus on during the waxing moon. They can be simple, one-time spells, or spells that we return to each night or day leading up to the full moon.

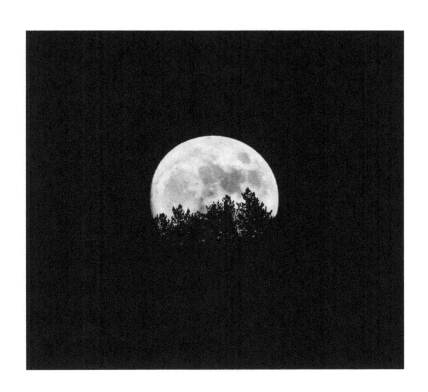

# The Full Moon Esbat

During a full moon esbat, the altar can be decorated in such a way as to honor the mother goddess or horned god.

- Items that represent the mother goddess, such as seashells, gourds, fresh flowers, eggs, cups of soil with seeds planted in them, honey, sweet cakes, meade, fruity wine, white grape juice, fresh water; items that represent the horned god, such as animal horns or skulls, crow feathers, a sword, a wooden staff, a crown, a cup made of stone or wood, whiskey, amber ale, red wine or grape juice.

- A statue or painting of either the horned god or the mother goddess (or both).

- Green, red, violet, gold, yellow or blue candles.

- The usual magical tools: chalice, athame, wand, and pentacle.

- An offering for the god or goddess, such as a cup of fresh water, bread, sweet cakes or cookies, sparkling wine or grape juice.

During a full moon esbat, one can focus on manifestation, abundance, self-love and readying oneself for love, life goals and dreams, healing, and spells to encourage strength and courage.

A full moon esbat is a wonderful time to raise magical vibrations that help the entire community, as well as the world. If you or your coven know of an area that has been affected by disaster or tragedy, sending healing and recovery energy their way during a full moon is a worthy practice.

During the full moon, we may focus on anything that needs the utmost energy. It can be things we wish to reach culmination (or release, such as finally getting good feedback on a project or hearing back from a job we applied for); it can be a simple matter of rejuvenating our inner selves after a difficult month, or sending healing energy to ourselves or others. The full moon is a time for recharging, so we set our tools and sacred objects out in the moon's light (or windowsill if you won't have access to a private space outdoors). Potions and elixirs we've created can be charged now, as well as amulets, sachets, and candles.

**There is actually no "wrong" time for magic.** Magic for pagans, including Wiccans, is merely a tool to help us focus our energy. If there is a need for magical work, don't let the phase of the moon deter you—it will simply result in the effects of your magic manifesting in a different way. A protection spell during a full moon may make the spell caster stronger, and less likely to feel the effects of who or what they're protecting themselves from; a protection spell during a waning moon will more likely push the source of the attack away or decrease the attack's potency.

A job search spell cast during a waning moon might actually cause you to *lose* your current job, but successfully find a new one during the coming days because you have more time to look. It's all a matter of perspective.

# Waning Moon

During a waning moon esbat, the altar can be decorated in such a way as to honor the crone.

- Items that represent the crone goddess. Keep in mind that the crone actually embodies all three aspects of the goddess, as she's lived through all three phases! Symbols of the triple goddess and triple moon can be placed on the altar, as well as the waning crescent moon, images in the colors of the sunset, midnight blue stones and artifacts, statues of owls, black cats, ravens, smoking pipes, copal incense, bundles of dried flowers and herbs, fruit cakes, meade, cider, port, black tea or coffee with sugar, fresh water, rice, and dried fruits.

- A statue or painting of either the crone goddess.

- Black, brown, dark red, midnight blue, silver, gray, or dark purple candles.

- The usual magical tools: chalice, athame, wand, and pentacle.

- An offering for the goddess, such as a cup of fresh water, bread, fruit cake, ale or cider, or sparkling grape juice.

The waning moon is quite important, also, and never to be thought of as negative. Sometimes, things need to wind down and to be let go of. The plants and flowers wilting and dying at the beginning of autumn feed the soil, and so does letting go of things which no longer serve us. During the waning moon, we can focus on the magic that releases anything in our lives that we need to let go of. It's a great time to do protection magic, as well as magic that supports getting rid of bad habits, weight loss, or the burden of shame, guilt, or any other negative emotion that is holding us back from happiness. The crone's wisdom at this time is like a loving great grandmother's—she wants us to succeed and to be joyful, so allow her to help you make your life so. During a waning moon esbat, spell work and rituals involving banishing and protection may be undertaken, as well as bidding goodbye to something or someone, and helping those in mourning deal with grief. It is a good time of the month for a memorial ceremony.

The waning moon is quite important and never to be thought of as negative. Sometimes, things need to wind down and to be let go of. The plants and flowers wilting and dying at the beginning of autumn feed the soil, and so does letting go of things which no longer serve us. During the waning moon, we can focus on the magic that releases anything in our lives that we need to let go of. It's a great time to do protection magic, as well as magic that supports getting rid of bad habits, weight loss, or the burden of shame, guilt, or any other negative emotion that is holding us back from happiness. The crone's wisdom at this time is like a loving great grandmother's—she wants us to succeed and to be joyful, so allow her to help you make your life so.

# The Dark Moon Esbat

This moon is also referred to as "the dead moon". It is a brief period of time when the moon is completely dark, showing that face to us on Earth while fully facing the sun. The dark moon is a good time for inner work and self-reflection, and so lends itself more to solitary observance than to a group or community magic.

Magic does not always have to be used to create a reaction—magic is the action, and the results of that magic can be considered the "reaction". There are times when sitting in a magic-filled space and contemplating the path ahead can be healing and affirming: the dark moon is one of the best times for this.

During a waning moon esbat, the altar can be decorated in such a way as to honor the crone or the elder god.

- Items that represent the crone, such as smoked teas, chicory coffee, grape juice or red wine, honey cakes or panettone, wreaths of ivy, hematite stones or smoky quartz; items that represent the elder god, such as mahogany, driftwood, pipe tobacco, dark ale, dark fruits or vegetables such as plums or purple peppers, petrified wood, amber, or granite.

- A statue or painting of either the elder god or the crone.

- Brown, gray, silver, or black candles.

- The usual magical tools: chalice, athame, wand, and pentacle.

- An offering for the god or goddess, such as a cup of fresh water, bread, seeded crackers, licorice or herbal candy, dark ale, grape juice, red wine.

Magic suitable for this esbat includes drawing love to you, as well as healing old wounds, overcoming obstacles, protection against theft and those who would stalk us, navigating divorce or separation, and help with addictions or injuries. The dark moon is a potent time for any divination, be it through the use of tarot cards, crystal ball or water scrying, runes, or simple candle magic.

# The Blue Moon Esbat

The blue moon occurs when two full moons happen in the same month. Blue moon energy is thought to be even more potent than full moon energy.

The folklore surrounding the blue moon tends to focus on luck and blessings:

- If you turn a coin in your pocket during this time, you gain tremendous luck and good fortune.

- gather plants beneath a blue moon for use in abundance and fortune spells

- Charge and bless objects to be used in magical work for finding a new job, bettering your finances, legal matters, and travel on your altar or outdoors beneath the lucky blue moon's light.

During the blue moon, the altar may be decorated to honor the god and the goddess in the aspect you feel most drawn to.

- Items that representing the masculine and the feminine of the natural world, hopes, dreams, luck, and good fortune may be placed there: rainbow items or stones, clover, crocus, basil and oregano, fresh flowers, crystal and pyrite, coins and paper money of each denomination, gold and silver, seashells and snail shells, rain and storm water, honey, champagne, cognac, cigars, fresh soil with seeds planted, amethyst, emeralds, and onyx. Blue flowers such as violet, iris, hydrangea, borage, and purple roses are also an excellent choice.

- A statue or painting of either the god and goddess or both.

- Candles in your favorite color, or a rainbow of colors. You may also choose to decorate the altar with blue items and use blue candles.

- The usual magical tools: chalice, athame, wand, and pentacle.

- An offering for the god or goddess, or both. A good choice is to have a potluck and fix one or two plates of the food served. Have additional bread, crackers, cookies, and either grape juice, water, or wine to pass around.

Magic suitable for this esbat include inciting change, growth, and healing, as well as love magic, financial spell work, money luck, and gambling luck, improved health and well-being.

**Purifying during a blue moon.** As a community or as a solitary practitioner, the blue moon presents a perfect opportunity for cleansing one's self spiritually. One might start by standing beneath the moon itself if the weather permits, allowing the healing energy to cast away any negativity or spiritual decay that's gathered on you from the previous month. Then return to the altar, cast your circle, and call down the energies of the moon. Music may be employed to set the mood. Take a bundle of healing herbs and ceremoniously trace them over the body—from head to feet—then burn them in a cauldron or bonfire to release the negativity.

**Make a list of goals for the future.** Take time during the blue moon to focus on your hopes and dreams for the coming months, and ask the goddess to grant you the insight, energy, and power to make those dreams come true. Make a note of this in your book of shadows so you can reflect on it in the coming months.

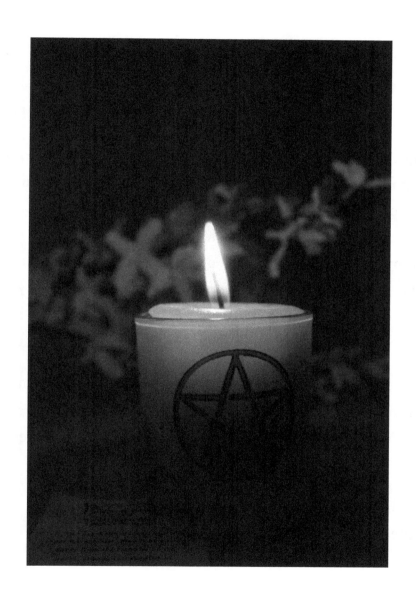

# Chapter 3: Magic and the Book of Shadows

## What Is Magic?

Magic, to pagans, is very real. There are many misconceptions about magic, however. The magic that Wiccans practice is not evil, not so-called "black" magic—it is simply a tool to help achieve a result. Just as prayer, meditation, exercise, and therapy are all tools to change one's path and one's thinking, so does magic work to help one navigate more successfully through life.

There are many different types of spells that can be performed, using a variety of materials. Before you get started on your first magic spell, however, it's important to do some research.

**The timing of spells.** As we discussed in the previous chapter, the phase of the moon is important, but also negotiable. It's best to time your spell work with the appropriate moon-phase, but if time is of the essence and the spell must be performed right away, then it can be done when you need to.

**Days of the week.** The days of the week also have magical significance. **Monday** is the day of the Moon, and good for beginnings, self-reflection, and healing. It is a mysterious day to work magic, so matters that are cut and dry are better left to other, more decisive days.

**Tuesday is a powerful day** and can lend itself well to matters of protection, finance, personal strength, and settling disputes in one's favor. Take care not to let your passions go to your head on this day, and strive to be peaceful in your affairs.

**Wednesday** is a good day for magic involving communication, career, getting the answers you've been waiting for, and expediting good news. Pray to the god Mercury, or to Ellegua—the trickster-messenger god of the Yoruba tribe—for aid in your work. Light incense and burn candles for Mercury to come swiftly. Offer Ellegua candies, cola, or a cigar for his help. Wearing red on Wednesday will bring good luck.

**Thursday** is a day ruled by Jupiter. It's a great day for spells regarding luck, prosperity, abundance, and beneficial change.

Offerings of wine, purple fruits and cakes to Jupiter with incense will help the god come around to your aid.

**Friday** is a day important in love and business. Many gods and goddesses call this day their own, such as Freya (after which the day is named), Oshun, Oya, Venus, and Erzulie. Spells for romantic matters, magical work to influence customers in the marketplace, and spells to be successful in court are all good things to focus on.

**Saturday** is ruled by Saturn, though it is also connected to Oshun the African love and riches goddess as well. Spells of protection, cleansing, personal strength, and wealth can be performed on this day.

**Sunday** is, of course, the day of the sun, and magic pertaining to vitality, good fortune, love, wealth, new beginnings can be performed on this day.

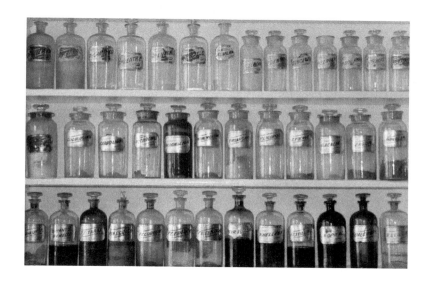

# Spell Components and the Magical Properties of Things

Now that you've selected the moon phase and day to perform your spell, what sort of things should you gather? A spell doesn't have to be complex unless you want it to be. Simple candle magic is incredibly effective, but so is herbal sachets and baths, herbal oils, and jar spells. Here are two lists to help you get started.

## *The magical significance of colors:*

- Blue: peace, healing, the mother goddess (such as Aphrodite or Yemaya), tranquility, wisdom. Use in spells for a peaceful home, fertility, and wisdom. Also good for helping one's psychic ability and communicating with angels.

- Green: fertility, growth, money magic, restorative magic, new beginnings, abundance. Use in spells for employment, good fortune, fertility.

- Yellow: communication, sexuality, attraction, intellectual matters, connection, magnetism. Use in spells for confidence, joyful sexuality, fertility, successful studies and high grades on tests, and communication.

- Orange: success, playful love, vitality, rejuvenation, energy. Use in spells for help with change, to enhance beauty and charisma, for success in one's craft, for confidence. Also a very good color for healing magic.

- Red: courage, strength in adversity, passionate love, health. Use in love spells, magic involving the power of will, and to enhance physical vitality.

- White: peace, mental balance, illumination, connection to ancestors, connection to the spirit world, blessing energy. Use to bless a space or a person, for a new home, to cleanse the spirit and body of negative energy, and for personal clarity.

- Black: protection, mysteries, banishing, binding, the wisdom of elders, fertility, stability. Use in spells for protection, banishing, transformation, and connecting to the elder god and crone goddess.

- Silver: psychic abilities, memory, clarity. Use for magic involving clairvoyance, creating a shield against negative energy, and spiritual awakening.

- Gold: the Sun god, past lives, intuitive powers, prosperity, new jobs, wealth. Use for money magic spells, spells for good luck, magic to connect to past life memories, and success.

- Brown: grounding energy, the Earth, fertility for the masculine, endurance, humble power. Use in magic for confidence, fertility, long-term financial success, a happy home, and for pets and other animals.

- Gray: self-reflection, neutrality, invisibility from one's enemies. Use in protection spells, neutralizing negative forces, understanding between two parties.

- Purple: wealth, luck, a rich life, delight, psychic powers, clairvoyant dreams. Use in spells to increase psychic ability, for good fortune, money magic, spiritual growth, connecting to angels and spirit guides, and self-control.

- Pink: romantic love, affection, youthfulness. Use in magic to remind oneself to find the beauty in things, for new romantic beginnings, magic for children.

## The magical significance of popular herbs and flowers:

- Acacia: protection, money magic, meditation, use in anointing candles and other magical objects. Also known as gum Arabic.

- Acorn: money magic, a happy home, amulets to promote youthful beauty, the wisdom of the elders and protection. Useful in luck magic.

- African violet: protection magic, lucky if kept in the home, good for the altar during Imbolc and Beltane.

- Apple: place on the altar during Samhain. Love spells, friendship, abundance.

- Basil: love, masculine energy, wealth, strength. Use in spells for a new job, success in business, and prosperity, as well as in love spells.

- Bay leaf: A super charge spells, luck, prosperity, protection, wishes coming true. Write a wish on a bay leaf and toss it in a fire to release your desire to the universe.

- Bayberry: good fortune, healing. Bayberry candles are excellent for money magic and to heal the heart.

- Carnation: spells of protection, inner strength, enhancing one's power in magic, ritual baths.

- Catnip: grown in one's garden or hung dried near the door, catnip protects the home.

- Cilantro: brings happy days to gardeners. Grown in the garden it will bring peace to the home.

- Cinnamon: luck, money, and passion. Use in spells to "heat up" the magic and expedite the results.

- Dandelion: divination, dreams, connecting to the spirit world. Use in sachets to help dreams come to fruition.

- Dragon's Blood: protection, cleansing. Burn to increase the potency of magical work. Carry for good luck.

- Echinacea: power, money, offerings to the spirits. Add to spells to boost their efficacy.

- Foxglove (poisonous to people and pets): beloved of fairies, protects the home as well as the garden. Grants visions.

- Frankincense: purification, noble endeavors, blessings.

- Garlic: protects the home and purifies spaces.

- Holly: joy in marriage, heightens masculinity, luck.

- Ivy: fertility magic, healing, protection against enemies.

- Job's tears: wishes comes true, blessings. Use in employment spells, mojo bags.

- Lavender: love, protection, peaceful heart. Helps with magical work to heal depression.

- Marjoram: purification magic, cleansing of spaces and self, used in sachets to attract wealth.

- Mint: helps businesses attract customers. Carry leaf in the wallet to ensure a constant flow of money in. Protects the home.

- Nutmeg: prosperity, money magic, luck. Use to break hexes.

- Oak: the tree regarded as most sacred. Use in fertility magic. Strength, wisdom, luck, vitality.

- Orange Blossoms: attraction, luck, money spells.
- Palo Santo: use to rid one's self and home from negative influences.

- Patchouli: love, money magic, luck.

- Rose: romantic and divine love, healing, avoiding negativity.

- Rosemary: sacred to faeries, ward against negativity, powerful banishing herb, and put in spells to boost power.

- Sage: traditionally used to cleanse a space. Also promotes healing, wisdom, and help with grief and mourning.

- Thyme: boosts reputation, hang in the home for protection and health.

- Vanilla bean: love and lust, increase magical abilities.

- Walnut: connection to the divine, blessings of the god and goddess, granting wishes.

# Preparing To Cast a Spell

Before you begin your magical work, make sure you prepare your space and yourself. You should have all of your ingredients and tools on hand. If you don't have a dedicated altar, a space on the floor that will be undisturbed by other people or pets will work fine. If you have time to take a ritual bath, that's great, but it's not essential.

When you're ready to begin, face the north. If you're unsure of where north is and do not have a compass, consider downloading a compass app for your phone, or look at an online map or surveyor's map of your property. You could also make note of where the sun rises and map the directions as such.

**Call the corners, or directions, to make your circle.**
You need a magical space that's filled with energy. You can't fill the entire world with your energy, so a circle gives you a dedicated space to work with. Start by facing north and saying Hail guardians of the north, I call to you in perfect love and trust." Then do so for each direction, turning clockwise (known as *sunwise* to Wiccans). Once you are done, say, the circle is cast." You are ready to begin your work.

---

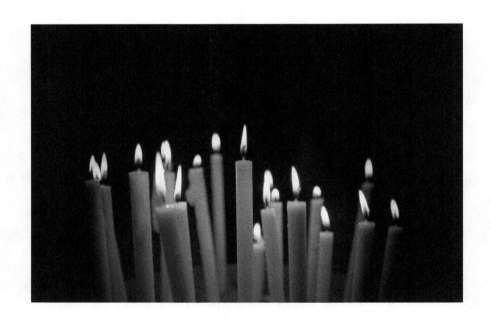

# A Simple Candle Spell

Select a candle in the appropriate color, and anoint it with oil in an appropriate herb or herbal mixture. Set this on your altar or temporary magical workspace, and light it. Light a stick of incense, and select a candle in the appropriate color, and anoint it with oil in an appropriate herb or herbal mixture. Set this on your altar or temporary magical workspace, and light it. Light a stick of incense, and draw sunwise circles in smoke around the candle as it burns. State what you would like to come true when the spell is complete; be specific. Imagine these things coming true like scenes in your mind. When you are ready, set the incense in a holder, and say, "I create this magic, to do as I say, to work for me both night and day. I create this magic by three times three, to harm no one else nor bring harm to me. I create this magic, so mote it be." Allow the candle to burn down to its finish. Never leave a candle unattended, but safe places for it to burn include a metal sink, metal pot or cauldron, or the bathtub. Make sure pets and small children will not have access to it.

# Full Moon Abundance Spell

This spell requires the power of the full moon; other moon phases will not be strong enough for the work to be successful. Gather a coin of every denomination; add to this a silver dollar, and a golden dollar. Fill a bowl, cauldron, or cup with rainwater and set it on your altar or magical workspace. Light two candles—use colors that represent the sun and the moon to you, and set them on either side of the container you are using.

Drop one coin into the water at a time, saying, Night and day, sun and moon, abundance coming to me soon, never stop, these coins I drop, night and day, sun and moon."

Set your container of water with the coins to bask in the full moon's light. The next day, set the coins on your altar, or gathers them in a cloth bag to a place near your workspace, wallet, or computer.

# One or the Other Candle Spell

If you have a question or two things you need to make a choice from, pick a candle in a color appropriate to your concern, and make sure it is not a dripless" candle. Set it on a dish, and place a nickel on one side of the candle, a penny on the other. Designate which coin represents which choice; if this is a simple yes or no question then the penny is yes and the nickel is no. Anoint the candle in rosemary, lavender, or simply olive oil and light it, focusing your mind on the choices in front of you. Speak your question, and ask the god and goddess to allow the candle to answer it for you.

Let the candle burn out until it's finished, and examine which coin has attracted the most wax: that is your answer.

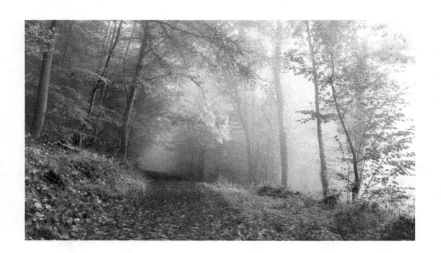

# Protection Spell for the Home

This can also be considered a spiritual cleansing" spell. Just like our carpets and our floors, our homes can get a lot of tracked in spiritual dirt", over time. After guests' visits or a repair person has come to fix the sink or just the simple act of you and your family coming home day after day, bringing with you the residual negativity of the outside world, it eventually will become necessary to sweep out the clutter so your unique, positive energy can shine through.

You'll want to gather four mason jars with lids that shut tight, some rice, lavender, and basil, as well as kosher salt for this spell.

**A note on spiritual cleansing.** Whether it's yourself, your house, a magical tool, or a piece of antique jewelry you found in a thrift store, mundane cleansing should always come before spiritual. Before you take a ritual bath, take a regular shower. Before you bless that vintage silver ring, polish it. Before you smudge your house, sweep it up, wipe the counters, and vacuum the rug. Doing this the day before sets your mind at ease so you can focus on your magical work.

Fill each jar with a handful of each ingredient. If you have a yard or outside space where neighbors won't pry, you can set each jar beside your house on each side, going from north to south. If you live in an apartment or flat or do not have private outside space, you can set a jar in a room that corresponds to each direction, at an exterior wall or on a windowsill.

As you set each jar down, say, North, south, east, and west, I ask you goddess, this house to bless." Let the jars remain a month and a day, then release the ingredients (toss in the garbage, in compost, or into the fire.)

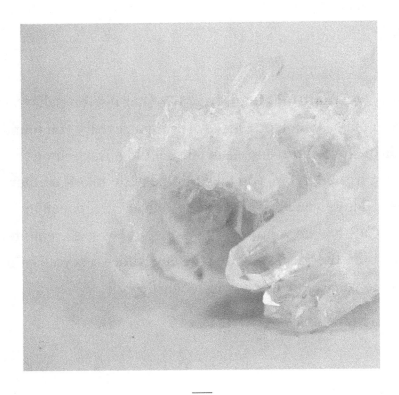

# Spells to Open Yourself to Love

**Love spells** are possibly the most common spells desired, aside from money spells.

You can find countless love spells promising to win someone's heart, rekindle cooled affections, trick someone into falling in love with you, sweeping someone off their feet, etc. What is the intention here? You might say, "to gain love".

What is the only foundation for true love? It's trust.

Recall the Wiccan tenet that we say in a circle and in performing spell work: "In perfect love and perfect trust." Love that is tricked into being will never be perfect or true. Love that is not based on trust is doomed to fail or fail again.

If you feel that you are ready to open yourself to a new romance, there is absolutely no reason not to do a magic spell to help you along with that. Consider it a pact with yourself to begin to be the loving, nurturing person you can be—and to also be willing to accept love from others.

These are just a few items that are useful in a love spell: rose petals, oil, or incense; rose quartz, hematite, amethyst, patchouli, rosemary, hibiscus, river stones (ask permission from the river goddess and spirits before taking one, and leave a gift of fruit or flowers at the riverbank), and Adam and Eve root (orchid root).

For roses, generally yellow petals mean friendship and platonic love, pink means new romantic love, and red means passionate love.

**A simple love spell is to cut halves of one red rose and one white rose,** tie them to make a single flower with string, then toss this charm into the water of a river, lake or waterfall, asking for love to come to you.

**Use rose oil** to anoint a white, pink, or red candle, and write the qualities of love you desire in a relationship. Fold the paper towards you three times and let the candle burn down upon it.

**Write down the qualities you seek in a romantic partner,** fold the paper towards you three times and bind with red string, then pin inside a red cloth. Keep this charm on you to attract the attention of new, true love.

**Carry a sprig of goldenrod** in your pocket to attract a love that will be both rejuvenating and secret (at first). Goldenrod is actually not a cause of allergies as many thinks, as its pollen does not become airborne.

**Take a ritual bath** in rose petals, a drop of patchouli oil, and set rose quartz in the water with you. Close your eyes and imagine a moment together with your true love. Repeat the words, God and goddess, them and me, at this moment, I will cry. In perfect love and perfect trust, allow destiny to join us." Allow the bathwater to drain but save a cup of it, along with the rose petals. Pat yourself dry gently, allowing the residual bathwater to remain on your skin. Toss the cup of water with petals in a crossroads, and true love will come your way in three months' time.

**Tell your secrets to the river goddess.** Place the river stone you found on your altar. Write down your hopes and dreams about love. Write down good qualities you find in yourself, and also challenges you've overcome and bad habits you've been able to put aside. Tell the goddess that you are ready for love to come into your life. Fold the paper three times towards you and place it beside the stone. Whenever you need a reminder that you are ready, gently hold the cool, smooth stone to your heart, and say, "Loving goddess, I am ready for the love that awaits me," as an affirmation.

# Honey Jars

**Rootwork** is a combination of many traditions and magical practices, coming over from Africa and the slave trade. Slaves in America needed to hide their magical work to avoid punishment, and began the tradition of using magic to survive in situations that were often dire. Today, rootwork exists as folk magic, and its nature is to be able to use what's on hand to produce extraordinary results. For a money, wealth, or abundance spell, write your very specific wishes on a piece of paper with a pencil, taking care not to lift the pencil off the paper until the statement is complete, fold it towards yourself twice, and place it in the jar with wealth-drawing herbs, shiny things of gold or silver, such as coins, gems, or biodegradable glitter. Seal the jar and burn gold, green, or silver candle on top for seven days, then three days during each full moon.

# Full Moon Abundance Spell

This spell requires the power of the full moon; other moon phases will not be strong enough for the work to be successful. Gather a coin of every denomination; add to this a silver dollar, and a golden dollar. Fill a bowl, cauldron, or cup with rainwater and set it on your altar or magical workspace. Light two candles—use colors that represent the sun and the moon to you, and set them on either side of the container you are using.

Drop one coin into the water at a time, saying, "Night and day, sun and moon, abundance coming to me soon, never stop, these coins I drop, night and day, sun and moon."

Set your container of water with the coins to bask in the full moon's light. The next days, set the coins on your altar, or gather them in a cloth bag to a place near your workspace, wallet, or computer.

## One or the Other Candle Spell

If you have a question or two things you need to make a choice from, pick a candle in a color appropriate to your concern, and make sure it is not a "dripless" candle. Set it on a dish, and place a nickel on one side of the candle, a penny on the other. Designate which coin represents which choice; if this is a simple yes or no question then the penny is yes and the nickel is no. Anoint the candle in rosemary, lavender, or simply olive oil and light it, focusing your mind on the choices in front of you. Speak your question, and ask the god and goddess to allow the candle to answer it for you.

Let the candle burn out until it's finished, and examine which coin has attracted the most wax: that is your answer.

## Protection Spell for the Home

This can also be considered a "spiritual cleansing" spells. Just like our carpets and our floors, our homes can get a lot of tracked in "spiritual dirt", over time. After guests visit or a repair person has come to fix the sink or just the simple act of you and your family coming home day after day, bringing with you the residual negativity of the outside world, it eventually will become necessary to sweep out the clutter so your unique, positive energy can shine through.

You'll want to gather four mason jars with lids that shut tight, some rice, lavender, and basil, as well as kosher salt for this spell.

**A note on spiritual cleansing.** Whether it's yourself, your house, a magical tool, or a piece of antique jewelry you found in a thrift store, mundane cleansing should always come before spiritual. Before you take a ritual bath, take a regular shower. Before you bless that vintage silver ring, polish it. Before you smudge your house, sweep it up, wipe the counters, and vacuum the rug. Doing this the day before sets your mind at ease so you can focus on your magical work.

Fill each jar with a handful of each ingredient. If you have a yard or outside space where neighbors won't pry, you can set each jar beside your house on each side, going from north to south. If you live in an apartment or flat or do not have private outside space, you can set a jar in a room that corresponds to each direction, at an exterior wall or on a windowsill.

As you set each jar down, say, North, south, east, and west, I ask you goddess, this house to bless." Let the jars remain a month and a day, then release the ingredients (toss in the garbage, in compost, or into the fire.)

# Spells to Open Yourself to Love

**Love spells** are possibly the most common spells desired, aside from money spells.

You can find countless love spells promising to win someone's heart, rekindle cooled affections, trick someone into falling in love with you, sweeping someone off their feet, etc. What is the intention here? You might say, "to gain love".

What is the only foundation for true love? It's trust.

Recall the Wiccan tenet that we say in a circle and in performing spell work: "In perfect love and perfect trust." Love that is tricked into being will never be perfect or true. Love that is not based on trust is doomed to fail or fail again.

If you feel that you are ready to open yourself to a new romance, there is absolutely no reason not to do a magic spell to help you along with that. Consider it a pact with yourself to begin to be the loving, nurturing person you can be—and to also be willing to accept love from others.

These are just a few items that are useful in a love spell: rose petals, oil, or incense; rose quartz, hematite, amethyst, patchouli, rosemary, hibiscus, river stones (ask permission from the river goddess and spirits before taking one, and leave a gift of fruit or flowers at the riverbank), and Adam and Eve root (orchid root).

For roses, generally yellow petals mean friendship and platonic love, pink means new romantic love, and red means passionate love.

**A simple love spell is to cut halves of one red rose and one white rose,** tie them to make a single flower with string, then toss this charm into the water of a river, lake or waterfall, asking for love to come to you.

**Use rose oil** to anoint a white, pink, or red candle, and write the qualities of love you desire in a relationship. Fold the paper towards you three times and let the candle burn down upon it.

**Write down the qualities you seek in a romantic partner**, fold the paper towards you three times and bind with red string, then pin inside a red cloth. Keep this charm on you to attract the attention of new, true love.

**Carry a sprig of goldenrod** in your pocket to attract a love that will be both rejuvenating and secret (at first). Goldenrod is actually not a cause of allergies as many thinks, as its pollen does not become airborne.

**Take a ritual bath** in rose petals, a drop of patchouli oil, and set rose quartz in the water with you. Close your eyes and imagine a moment together with your true love. Repeat the words, "God and goddess, they and I, at this moment, I will scry. In perfect love and perfect trust, allow destiny to join us." Allow the bathwater to drain but save a cup of it, along with the rose petals. Pat yourself dry gently, allowing the residual bathwater to remain on your skin. Toss the cup of water with petals in a crossroads, and true love will come your way in three months' time.

**Tell your secrets to the river goddess.** Place the river stone you found on your altar. Write down your hopes and dreams about love. Write down good qualities you find in yourself, and also challenges you've overcome and bad habits you've been able to put aside. Tell the goddess that you are ready for love to come into your life. Fold the paper three times towards you and place it beside the stone. Whenever you need a reminder that you are ready, gently hold the cool, smooth stone to your heart, and say, "Loving goddess, I am ready for the love that awaits me," as an affirmation.

# Honey Jars

**Rootwork** is a combination of many traditions and magical practices, coming over from Africa and the slave trade. Slaves in America needed to hide their magical work to avoid punishment, and began the tradition of using magic to survive in situations that were often dire. Today, rootwork exists as folk magic, and its nature is to be able to use what's on hand to produce extraordinary money, wealth, or abundance spell, write your very specific wishes on a piece of paper with a pencil, taking care not to lift the pencil off the paper until the statement is complete, fold it towards yourself twice, and place it in the jar with wealth-drawing herbs, shiny things of gold or silver, such as coins, gems, or biodegradable glitter. Seal the jar and burn gold, green, or silver candle on top for seven days, then three days during each full moon.

# Grimoire or Book of Shadows

Your book of shadows is a place for you to compile the spell work you do, your observations during magical work, and inspirations, prophetic dreams, or anything else that you experience on your path in Wicca. It should be kept sacred to you, and private. Avoid using it as a mundane journal, and do not include negative spell work in its pages.

**Black vs. White magic.** Some say that white magic is ineffective and that so-called "black" magic is anything that works. Recall how the words black and dark are not negative; they're part of the natural world (as well as part of our human world). So, instead of using words of color to discuss magic, let's focus on *intent*. Your intention is what carries through your magic on the tides of your will. If you have harmful intentions, it's best to focus on self-healing and reflection. Life is full of challenges, and sometimes we might be tempted to use our magical knowledge for revenge or to sway someone else to our side.

Magic aimed at another person is simply not the Wiccan way. Recall the Rede: "and it harm none, do what ye will." Think about this tenet each time you begin to plan a new magical work, for whatever you put into the world returns to you, threefold.

# Chapter 4: Solitary vs. Coven

## The Solitary Witch

Of the many traits and sensibilities Wiccans, as well as pagans, have in common; a stubborn streak of individuality exists. This is perhaps what makes a witch, a witch—the will to do as they will, that it harm none, in their own, unique way. Because of this independence, many Wiccans choose to practice their faith alone. There is a beauty in connecting to nature and the gods on one's own terms, following a path that they alone can hear. In this role, the new witch is very much a student, and the entire universe, their teacher. Even Wiccans with decades-long experience, however, can find peace and meaning as a solitary practitioner.

## The Coven

That being said, joining together with one's community can be a heady experience indeed. Group ceremony can be extraordinarily moving and affirming. Rites of passage such as initiation, wiccaning, naming, hand-fasting, and croning are celebratory moments that a close-knit, trusted community will gather around and add to the personal joy of the celebrant and initiate.

**Finding a coven** can be tricky, however, and finding an earnest group of folks that you bond with, time-consuming. A coven can be quite large in these modern times, but it can also be a small group. In the latter case, the personalities have to match each other, and not clash. A good place to start if you're looking for a coven is a pagan community group—not officially a coven, but a group of like-minded folks who come together to celebrate the sabbats and esbats. Social media and the internet is a great place to start looking for local communities near you. When you find their websites, read what they're the focus is: some groups devote themselves to worshipping the goddess only while others follow both the goddess and the god. Some are for adults only, others are all ages. Once you start attending a few public circles and get to know some of the people there, you may get insight into where to find an established coven that are looking for new members.

# Conclusion

Thank for making it through to the end of *Wicca for Beginners*, let's hope it was informative and able to provide you with all of the tools you need to achieve your goals whatever they may be.

The next step is to look at the natural world around you. How do you see yourself in it? In what ways do you see the god and goddess in the world? The best way to begin your Wiccan path is to realize that you are a part of the world, and it is a part of you.

Finally, if you found this book useful in any way, a review on Amazon is always appreciated!